THE FEMMEPHOBIA 101
Workbook

By: Rhea Ashley Hoskin, Toni Serafini, Jocelyne Scott, & Karen L. Blair (2023)

Illustrated by Cindy Zhang

Copyright Year: 2023

Copyright Notice: by Rhea Ashley Hoskin, Toni Serafini, Jocelyne Scott & Karen L. Blair. All rights reserved.

The above information forms this copyright notice: © 2023 by Rhea Ashley Hoskin, Toni Serafini, Jocelyne Scott & Karen L. Blair. All rights reserved.

ISBN: 978-1-312-75136-1

OVERVIEW

① **WELCOME**
pp. 5-6

② **EXPLORING FEMININITY**
pp. 7-10

③ **THE GENDER BINARY**
pp. 11-12

④ **EXPLORING FEMME**
pp. 13-18

⑤ **FEMME THEORY**
pp. 19-21

⑥ **FEMMEPHOBIA**
pp. 22-29

⑦ **GENDER-BASED OPPRESSION**
pp. 30-37

⑧ **THE "RULES" OF FEMININITY**
pp. 38-47

⑨ **STOPPING FEMMEPHOBIA**
pp. 48-55

⑩ **TAKE AWAYS**
pp. 56-58

⑪ **FINAL REFLECTIONS**
pp. 59-60

⑫ **RESOURCES**
pp. 62-65

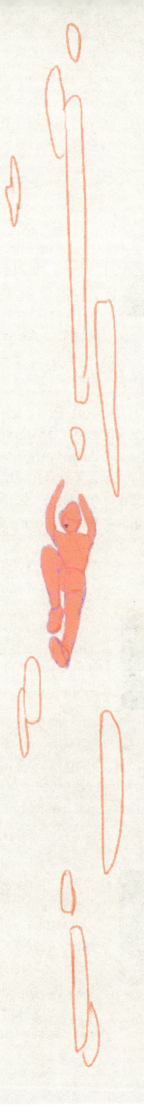

WORKBOOK AUTHORS

Meet your authors! For more information on how to contact us, see page 61

DR. RHEA ASHLEY HOSKIN

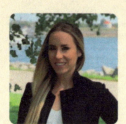

Rhea Ashley Hoskin is an interdisciplinary feminist sociologist whose work focuses on Critical Femininities, Femme Theory, and femmephobia. Her work examines perceptions of femininity and sources of prejudice rooted in the devaluation and regulation of femininity. Dr. Hoskin is an AMTD Global Talent Postdoctoral Fellow and SSHRC Postdoctoral Fellow at the University of Waterloo and St. Jerome's, where she is cross-appointed to the departments of Sociology & Legal Studies, and Sexuality, Marriage, & Family Studies.

DR. JOCELYNE SCOTT

Jocelyne Bartram Scott, Ph.D. (she/her) is the Director of Equity and Inclusive Excellence at Bucknell University. Prior to her appointment at Bucknell University she worked within Women's and Gender Studies and student retention services at Texas Tech University and Indiana University. She uses her expertise in feminist and queer theory, critical race theory, and critical femininity studies to create research-based diversity, equity, and inclusion interventions.

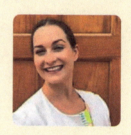

DR. KAREN BLAIR

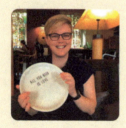

Dr. Karen L. Blair is an Associate Professor of Psychology at Trent University. She is the Director of the KLB Research Lab and the Trent University Social Relations, Attitudes, and Diversity Lab. Her research focuses on LGBTQ psychology, social support, relationships and health, prejudice, femmephobia, hate crimes, and Holocaust education.

CINDY ZHANG

Cynthia (Cindy) Zhang is a Forensic Biology major at Trent University, and an artist with a keen interest in science-fiction and visual development, pursuing professional illustration and design alongside their studies.

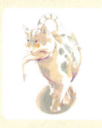

DR. TONI SERAFINI

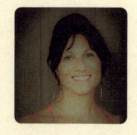

Dr. Toni Serafini (she/they) is an Associate Professor and former Chair of the Department of Sexuality, Marriage, and Family Studies at St. Jerome's University (@UWaterloo). Her teaching and research unite around intersectional, feminist, and anti-oppressive practices and pedagogies. Some of her current projects include exploring bodies as identity markers and the development of a measure of femmephobia (with Dr. Hoskin). Toni is also a Registered Psychotherapist and relational therapist with a small private practice.

ABOUT THIS WORKBOOK

What comes to mind when you think about femininity?

When you meet a feminine person, what assumptions do you make about them?

What assumptions do you feel others make about your femininity?

Have you ever tried to distance yourself from feminine things, traits, or people?

In this workbook you will learn to identify the rules, expectations, and assumptions about femininity and who they impact. By considering whose femininity is accepted by society and the limits society places on femininity, we hope this workbook will help you embrace feminine diversity and build an understanding of the broader impact of femmephobia (i.e., the way society devalues and regulates femininity).

We will discuss the role and impact of femmephobia in our daily lives and help you to brainstorm how to interrupt femmephobia in ourselves and others through everyday actions. Ultimately, through this workbook we hope you will better understand the relationship between gender-based oppression and femmephobia. Together, we will learn the importance of understanding femmephobia to make our communities, families, and relationships places where we can all be ourselves - whatever that looks like. In this workbook, we will examine concepts such as femininity, femme, femme theory, and femmephobia. Throughout the workbook, we will ask you to reflect on your own feelings and experiences related to femininity.

Content in this workbook was first developed for the purpose of workshops on femmephobia. By turning our workshop into a workbook, we hope to reach more people and start broader conversations about the treatment of femininity in our social world and relationships.

Please note that all word clouds and examples are composites generated by members of the research team through our previous research, knowledge of the community, and personal experiences. No participant data are shared in this workbook, other than those previously published in other work.

WELCOME!

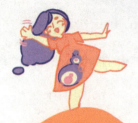

The meanings we assign to things vary from person to person - not all of us see or understand the world in the same way. The following reflective activities invite you to think about your personal views, beliefs, and how you make sense of the world around you. As such, there are no right or wrong answers.

While we start this workbook with reflection exercises, there is no correct order to work through this book. You may find that answering some of the questions is difficult without reading through the entire workbook. This workbook is intended for you, and your personal journey examining and unlearning femmephobia. As such, we invite you to use the workbook in whatever way or order makes the most sense for you.

Flip forward, flip backward, or progress through the material as we've laid it out.

WHAT IS FEMININITY?

Write down the first 5 words or phrases that come to mind when you hear or read the term "femininity"?

1. _____
2. _____
3. _____
4. _____
5. _____

What are some stereotypes, assumptions, myths, or tropes about femininity and feminine people?

_____

SELF-REFLECTION

Everyone has a relationship to femininity, no matter their sex (assigned at birth), gender, or sexual orientation.

How would you describe your relationship with femininity?

_____
_____
_____
_____
_____
_____
_____
_____

Think about periods in your life that may have marked a change in this relationship - what was happening at that time that may have impacted your relationship with femininity?

_____
_____
_____
_____
_____
_____
_____
_____

Similarly, our relationships with certain people or events/experiences can shape our relationship to femininity. What stands out for you when you think of the people or events that shaped your relationship to femininity?

_____
_____
_____
_____
_____
_____
_____
_____

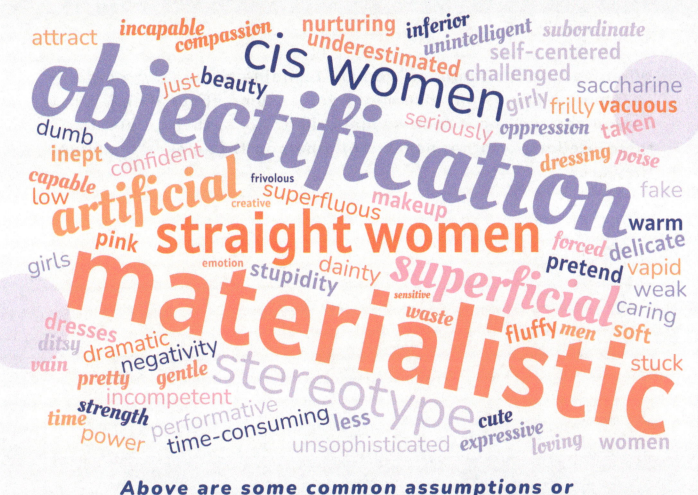

Above are some common assumptions or stereotypes relating to femininity.

When you look at these words or phrases, what stands out for you? What do you notice? How do they fit with your own ideas, beliefs, and values (or not)?

_____
_____
_____
_____
_____
_____
_____
_____
_____
_____
_____
_____

SELF-REFLECTION

When you meet a feminine woman, feminine nonbinary* person, or feminine man, what else might you assume about them? What do you assume about their sexual orientations, their interests, their intellect, or other aspects of a person that makes them who they are?

A feminine woman is:
_____
_____
_____
_____
_____
_____
_____

A feminine man is:
_____
_____
_____
_____
_____
_____
_____

A feminine nonbinary person is:
_____
_____
_____
_____
_____
_____
_____

*A nonbinary person refers to someone who does not identify as being a "man" or a "woman." Sometimes they identify as both, sometimes they identify as neither.

THE GENDER BINARY

Everyone makes assumptions and judgments all the time! It's a necessary part of how our brains process the world around us. Sometimes the shortcuts we make in trying to understand others can reflect biased assumptions. Some of these shortcuts relate to the gender binary. The gender binary is a cultural belief that there are only two genders: man and woman. Within this belief system, men are supposed to be masculine, and women are to be feminine.

What things come to mind when you think about:

MASCULINE APPEARANCE

FEMININE APPEARANCE

MASCULINE BEHAVIOUR

FEMININE BEHAVIOUR

MASCULINE PEOPLE

FEMININE PEOPLE

NOW, LET'S UNPACK THIS...

What was the experience of filling in those boxes like for you?
What did you notice about yourself when you were thinking about what to write?
What was difficult and what was easy?

_____
_____
_____
_____
_____
_____
_____
_____

When you look back at the lists you created, what are some of the assumptions or biases that may have shaped your responses? How did the gender binary and the belief that there are only two genders limit or direct/shape your responses?

For example, it is probably difficult to answer the question about feminine appearance or behaviour without listing some 'stereotypical feminine' things, like squealing, clapping hands, having a high voice, wearing make-up/nail polish, and so on. How do these behaviours or appearances connect to being feminine? Can a feminine person have a lower voice? Not wear make-up? Be a man?

_____
_____
_____
_____
_____
_____
_____
_____

WHAT IS FEMME?

If you are unsure, feel free to return to this page later after viewing the rest of the book.

What does femme mean to you?

_____
_____
_____
_____
_____
_____
_____
_____

What assumptions do you make about <u>femme</u> people? In what ways do they differ from your assumptions about <u>feminine</u> people, if any?

_____
_____
_____
_____
_____
_____
_____
_____
_____
_____
_____
_____

The word cloud below contains some words and phrases to describe femme, along with some common assumptions or stereotypes about femmes.

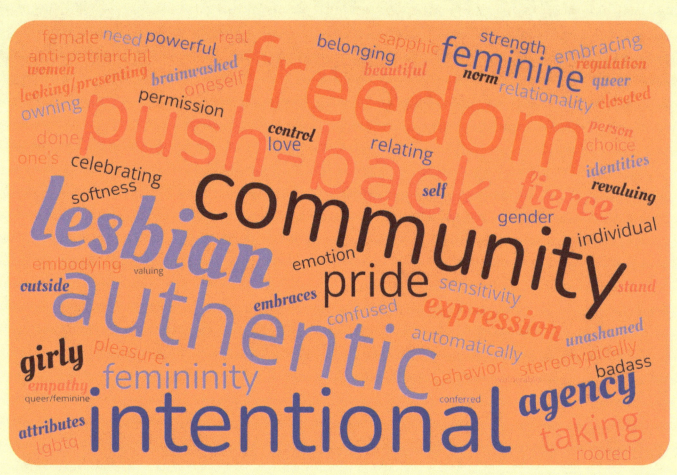

When you look at these words or phrases, what stands out for you? What do you notice? How do they fit with your own ideas, beliefs, and values (or not)?

_____
_____
_____
_____
_____
_____
_____
_____
_____
_____

FEMME & FEMININITY

At the beginning of the workbook, you were asked to reflect on your beliefs and assumptions about **femininity**. Then, you were asked to reflect on your beliefs and assumptions about **femmes**.

What do you notice about the similarities and differences between the two lists?

FEMME HISTORY

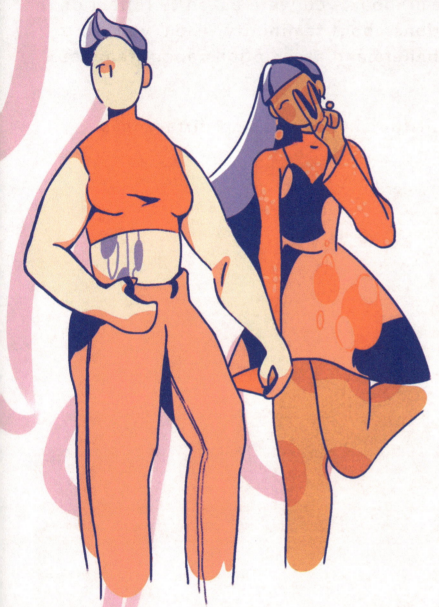

The term "femme" came from 1940s/50s working-class lesbian bar cultures where "femmes" (feminine lesbians) coupled with "butches" (masculine lesbians) (see Kennedy & Davis, 1993; Nestle, 1992).

While 'femme' will always have roots in lesbian communities and cultures, this term has grown and expanded significantly since the late-20th century.

We see these changes within LGBTQ+* communities themselves, and also in academic research.

For instance, in their research, Karen Blair & Rhea Ashley Hoskin (2015; 2016) found that femme is an identity that resonates across genders and sexualities, including cisgender and transgender women and men, nonbinary people, and people of all sexual orientations. So "femme" is not just for feminine lesbians anymore!

...SO WHAT DOES FEMME MEAN NOW?

*LGBTQ+ refers to lesbian, gay, bisexual, transgender, queer people, and all of the many identities that expand beyond heterosexual and cisgender. In Turtle Island/North America, we often start this acronym with "2S," meaning Two-Spirit. However, this term is typically reserved for the Indigenous people of Turtle Island. Because there are so many "LGBTQ+" Indigenous identities outside of Western contexts, it may not be appropriate to apply Two-Spirit outside of Western contexts.

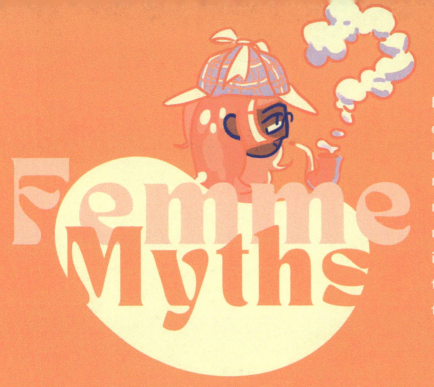

Femme Myths

Before we tackle the big question of "what does femme mean now," let's do some myth-busting. There are so many myths and misconceptions about femme identities that it is impossible to list them all! We've picked three:

1. Gaydar: People can "look gay"

The way someone looks has little to do with their sexual identity or attractions. Sure, sometimes our assumptions turn out to be right - but this is what researchers call "confirmation bias" and the "representativeness heuristic," both help to maintain the idea (myth) that a person LOOKS gay or straight (i.e., feminine men are assumed to be gay, and masculine women are assumed lesbians). Yes, a feminine man MIGHT be gay ... but gay men can be masculine, too! Masculine men just never catch our eye as being potentially gay. And actually, not every feminine man is gay. In fact, statistically, most feminine men are straight!

We know that there are so many aspects of sexual and gender diversity that things can sometimes get muddy. Let's clear this up a bit! People of all gender identities can express femininity, masculinity, and androgyny, and this has little to do with their sexual orientation (or even gender identity!). These things are separate, but we often mash them all together. Stopping this way of thinking from seeping into our language and assumptions helps many people both within and outside LGBTQ+ communities!

Confirmation Bias
When you only pay attention to information that helps you believe something that you already think is true, and you don't pay attention to information that might tell you're wrong.

Representativeness Heuristic
When you make decisions about things based on how similar they seem to a typical example or stereotype, even if you don't have all the information you need.

2. Femmes are brainwashed or anti-feminist

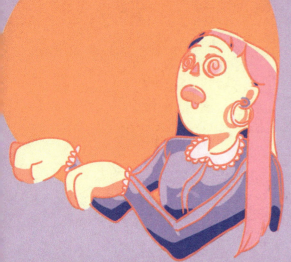

Femmes have a long history of being seen as anti-feminist, and have not always been welcome within feminist groups! Here, and within broader society, femmes are sometimes seen as being "brainwashed" by society to be feminine. History lesson aside, many femmes ARE feminists and CHOOSE to 'lean into' expressing their femininity openly and with pride because their femininity is an important part of who they are.

3. Femme lesbians use their femininity to hide their sexual orientation

It is common for people to think that femme lesbian women are "in the closet" and trying to hide their sexual orientation, or that they are somehow less "out" than butch lesbians or more masculine queer and bisexual women. Bisexual and queer femmes are also seen as less "authentically queer." These are both based on the assumption or false belief that all feminine women are straight. Femmes are seen as "using" this assumption to their advantage as a way to hide their sexuality. But for many femmes, this could not be further from the truth! In fact, we know that femmes have historically wanted to be seen and accepted as BOTH femme and lesbian or bisexual.

This is still the case today, as seen in the research by Gunn and colleagues (2021) and Blair and Hoskin (2015; 2016). There were no differences in how "out" femme, butch, or androgynous women were - so being "feminine" or "masculine" had nothing to do with trying to hide their sexual orientation (or their internalized homophobia, for that matter).

FEMME IDENTITY VS. FEMME THEORY

Now that we've busted some myths, let's tackle the big question of **what femme means today!**

While there are as many different definitions of femme as there are femmes, some femme scholars have defined "femme" as femininity reclaimed by queer and culturally marginalized folks (Hoskin, 2021b). In other words, femme is femininity by people who aren't usually **allowed to be feminine** (e.g., lesbian women or men), and/or who **don't fit the norms of "acceptable" femininity** (e.g., fat or disabled people).

These norms also include who femininity is for and how it should be experienced or expressed (e.g., expressed by women for the purpose of attracting men).

Femme theory originated from the perspectives of femmes and their experiences of having their femininity controlled, regulated, and devalued. Those perspectives were applied in such a way that FEMME THEORY was born!

But how do they identify? Looking or behaving feminine doesn't make someone femme.

Remember to never assume anything about someone's identity based on appearance - femmes included!

... they look super femme.

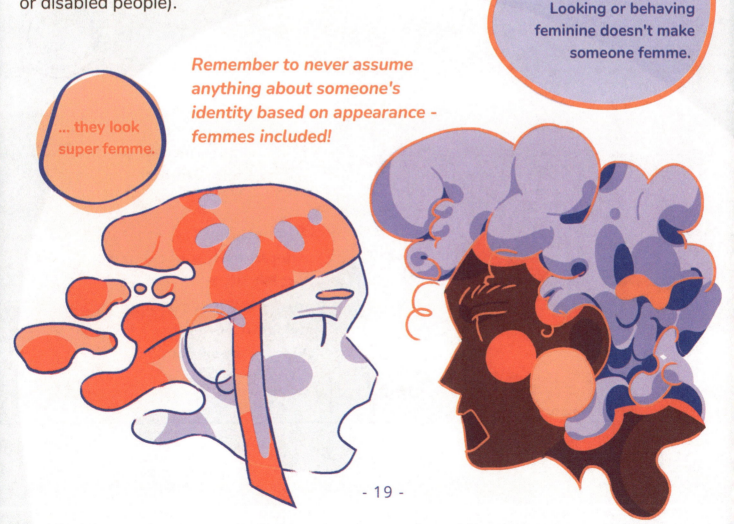

What does Femme Theory "do"?

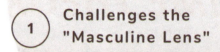

1. Challenges the "Masculine Lens"

Masculinity is the "lens" we tend to look through to see and evaluate the world around us. The masculine lens thus shapes where and how we place value - we value things seen as masculine and, in turn, devalue things seen as feminine. If we reverse the focus and place femininity at the centre, femme theory helps us to **see** this "taken-for-granted" masculine value system.

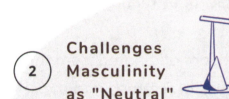

2. Challenges Masculinity as "Neutral"

Because of this tendency to view the world through a "masculine lens," we also tend to see masculinity as the default (or norm). In other words, we see masculinity as "gender neutral" because masculinity and men are not only considered superior but are also often the "default" of gender expression and gender identity. A good example of this is how society is more comfortable with a woman (gender identity) wearing pants (gender expression) than a man (gender identity) wearing a skirt (gender expression). This imbalance is, in part, a product of seeing masculinity as neutral.

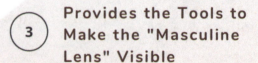

3. Provides the Tools to Make the "Masculine Lens" Visible

If something is taken-for-granted as the norm or as natural (like masculinity), how can we even begin to notice its presence? For this, **we need femme theory!**

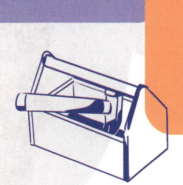

WHAT'S IN THE "FEMME THEORY" TOOLBOX?

One of these tools is the concept of "femmephobia"

WHAT IS FEMMEPHOBIA?

When you hear/see the word 'femmephobia,' what comes to mind?

Femmephobia refers to the devaluation and regulation of femininity or the way that femininity is seen as "lesser than," sometimes rejected, and often scrutinized by others within society.

Hoskin (2017;2020)

Identifying Femmephobia

Examples of femmephobia can be found <u>everywhere</u> - across different groups, identities, and experiences.

What are some examples of femmephobia in LGBTQ+ communities?

_____
_____
_____
_____
_____
_____
_____
_____
_____

What are some examples of femmephobia outside of LGBTQ+ communities (e.g., sports, the workplace, politics, pop culture)?

_____
_____
_____
_____
_____
_____
_____
_____
_____
_____
_____
_____

The Feminine Joke

One form of femmephobia is "the feminine joke."
Let's break that down!

Have you ever noticed that femininity is used to mock or ridicule political leaders? Or perhaps you've noticed that femininity is sometimes the punchline or the brunt of a joke? On Saturday Night Live or scrolling through Instagram, viewers roll with laughter at the sight of a man in make-up or a dress. Sometimes we even use this "feminine joke" to mock men in power (e.g., Donald Trump, Vladimir Putin) and to "take them down a notch," so to speak.

We see the feminine joke subtly and not-so-subtly throughout the day, and typically give it little thought or attention - because using femininity to "poke fun" at someone happens all the time (e.g., feminizing sports teams or athletes by calling them "princesses").

But why is this funny? Why and how does femininity "take down" men in power? And how might treating femininity in this way contribute to other forms of gender-based oppression, such as sexism/misogyny, homophobia, and transphobia (see page 31)?

Whether we're using femininity to demote, mock, or "entertain," the feminine joke keeps femininity as something that's seen as "lesser." As a result, we take feminine people less seriously and see them as less credible, less competent, less authentic, and less powerful.

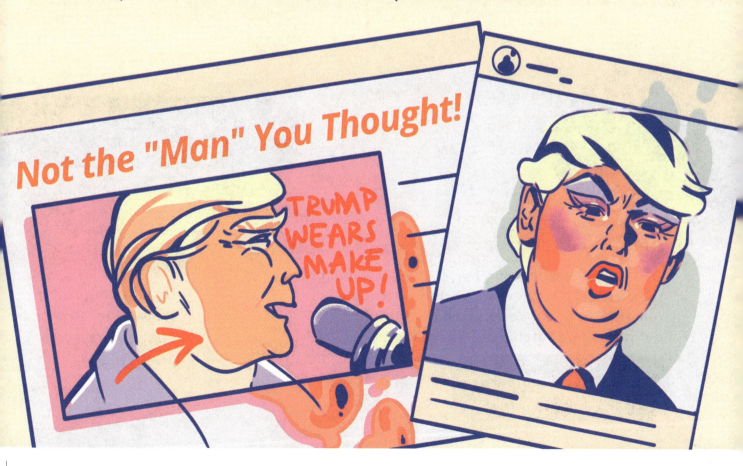

MORE EXAMPLES OF FEMMEPHOBIA

Femmephobia takes many forms - it can be opinions we hold or experiences we have had...or both! Femmephobia can target how a person dresses, the way they speak, their mannerisms, and so on. Below are some examples of femmephobia:

Wow, she's asking for it with that skirt!

Try to "tone it down" a bit if you want to be taken seriously...

To be honest, I can't take feminine women in STEM fields seriously.

Last night I was at the bar and I was literally glared at and asked why I was there. Then in the morning I went to class and had my gender studies professor use the term "look straight" to refer to femmes!

I'd be fine if my kid was a tomboy... but I can't handle a sissy.

She's such a girly girl - it's very annoying.

Why do we use femininity to mock political leaders like Trump, Putin, Jong-un or others? Why do we find this funny?

"No, men can't get Pumpkin Spice lattes, a black coffee maybe haha"

Don't wear a dress if you want to be taken seriously.

When feminine individuals are devalued or seen as being not as smart.

Trans men need to reject femininity if they want to "pass" ... you know, to be real men.

Your emotions make you weak!

No fats, no femmes, no Asians!

Masc only!

Intelligent people don't bother with makeup.

I don't care if you're gay... just don't be a fairy.

More feminine presenting women cannot be queer and are always straight and just looking for attention.

Feminine women who claim to be nonbinary are just after attention.

Don't wear heels to the bar, but always wear them to job interviews...but don't act too feminine or you'll seem incompetent and definitely less intelligent!

Ugh, straight women in queer spaces are so annoying.

I'm not like other girls...

APPLICATIONS IN RESEARCH

If you didn't know it before this workbook, femmephobia is a REAL THING, and there is research to prove it!

Femme Theory and the concept of femmephobia have been used to analyze:

- DATING & RELATIONSHIPS
- MASK-WEARING BEHAVIOUR DURING COVID-19
- BEAUTY PRACTICES
- FASHION & AESTHETICS
- POP CULTURE

- GENDER-BASED VIOLENCE (INCLUDING HOMOPHOBIA, TRANSPHOBIA, SEXUAL VIOLENCE, ETC.)
- FITNESS CULTURE
- BREASTFEEDING
- THE MILITARY

- INCEL IDEOLOGY
- EDUCATION & PEDAGOGY
- FAT BODIES & FATPHOBIA
- WORKPLACE HARASSMENT
- ENVIRONMENT
- SPORTS

- BODY IMAGE & DISORDERED EATING
- GENDER & LABOUR
- MENTORSHIP
- FAMILIES

... and so much more!

IMPACT OF FEMMEPHOBIA

As you can see, femmephobia takes many forms and is always directed at devaluing feminine expressions while regulating who can BE feminine, when, where, how, and so on.
So, who are the people that femmephobia impacts?

Femmephobia can impact more than individual people. When you think about social structures, systems, and processes (e.g., education, healthcare, law, families), *how do you see femmephobia working? How does it impact those larger forces?*

WHO DOES FEMMEPHOBIA IMPACT?

WHO?

- Women
- Men
- Nonbinary people
- All sexual orientations and identities
- Feminine AND masculine people!

WHAT DOES THIS MEAN?

- Femmephobia limits who is allowed to be feminine and in what ways.
- As a result, femmephobia limits the freedom people have to express themselves.

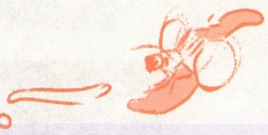

If we take a moment, each of us can probably think of times when we have seen or experienced femmephobia – regardless of our gender identity (woman, man, nonbinary), sex assigned at birth (female, male, intersex), sexual identity (lesbian, gay, bisexual, asexual), or how feminine/masculine we are in our dress, voice, mannerisms, interests, and so on. We have all seen, made, or experienced negative comments about feminine traits, behaviours, and expressions (e.g., "drama queen"). Most of us live in societies that place a high value on masculinity and things considered "masculine" (e.g., strength, control, competence, a certain way of dressing/acting). Because of this, we experience pressures to "be masculine" and "be feminine" in very specific, prescribed (or controlled) ways – all based on our assumed sex, age, body size, race, and class (among other personal traits). The "rules" for when and how to be feminine or masculine can change from context to context (e.g., family, work, school) and person-to-person - different rules at different ages, for different races/bodies/genders. There is no "one size fits all" for "acceptable femininity"! And that's because femininity is controlled or regulated ... more on this later!

GENDER-BASED OPPRESSION

Gender-based oppression refers to the different types of prejudice, discrimination, oppression, and violence that can connect to gender or the way people are seen as "expressing" gender. Below are examples of gender-based oppression, including, but not limited to, sexism, misogyny, transphobia, homophobia, and femmephobia.

These terms may be new to you, somewhat familiar but confusing, or maybe you know them well! Whatever your current knowledge, take a stab at connecting the "term" on the left to the definition on the right:

SEXISM/MISOGYNY	Targets femininity or perceived femininity in all people - across gender and sexual identities.
TRANSPHOBIA	Targets people who are perceived to be lesbian or gay.
HOMOPHOBIA	Targets people who do not follow the "rules" for their assigned sex (e.g., female/male) and gender (e.g., how to be a woman or a man, according to the gender binary).
FEMMEPHOBIA	Targets people for being female or a woman.

Check your answers on the next page!

TEASING APART DIFFERENT TYPES OF GENDER-BASED OPPRESSION

1 — **Femmephobia** targets femininity or perceived femininity in all people - across gender and sexual identities.

2 — **Homophobia** targets people who are perceived to be lesbian or gay. Assumptions about sexuality often connect to the gender binary and femmephobia, but these prejudices (homophobia and femmephobia) are different.

3 — **Transphobia** targets people who do not follow the "rules" for their assigned sex (e.g., female/male) and gender (e.g., how to be a woman or a man, according to the gender binary). This can relate to femininity, and often does, but not always.

4 — **Sexism and misogyny** target people for being female or a woman. While that sometimes overlaps with femininity, they're not the same - a woman can be feminine, but she can also be masculine or androgynous. We need specific terms to be able to talk about each dimension.

Femmephobia weaves through each of these gender-based prejudices and offers us new ways to tackle them.

Femmephobia, Sexism/Misogyny & Homophobia

How does femmephobia relate to and/or differ from sexism and misogyny?

How does femmephobia relate to and/or differ from homophobia?

How does femmephobia relate to and/or differ from transphobia?

WOMEN ARE COMPLEX

As are men and nonbinary people, of all sexual orientations!

Looking back at 1940s butch/femme communities, we have examples of how women can be feminine, masculine, or anywhere in between. Of course, men and nonbinary people can also be feminine or masculine.

Because it can be a bit tricky to separate misogyny and sexism from femmephobia, one way to help is to think back to butch/femme lesbian communities and remember that...

All people, including women, can be:

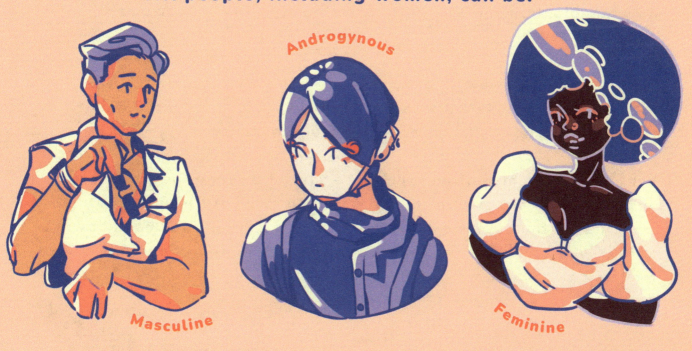

Masculine — Androgynous — Feminine

But only women experience sexism and misogyny because they target a person's gender/sex.

FEMMEPHOBIA, on the other hand, **focuses on femininity, and all genders** - women, men, nonbinary people - **can be feminine** (or masculine, or androgynous). Because everyone can be feminine, femmephobia is something that targets and can be experienced **by all bodies, genders, and sexual orientations.**

RECAP: FEMMEPHOBIA

A UNITING FRAMEWORK FOR GENDER-BASED VIOLENCE

The relationship between femmephobia and other forms of gender-based oppression can be confusing!

A good analogy for understanding this relationship is to think about femmephobia as a linking chain that weaves throughout various types of gender-based violence and oppression, including sexism/misogyny, homophobia, transmisogyny (transphobia aimed at trans women), and more!

While not all or always, many forms of violence connected to gender can be traced to femininity and feminine expressions - and the fact that society tends to devalue and control femininity.

For example, women often experience sexism through the treatment and regulation of their femininity, gay (and straight!) men are targeted for their femininity, and our idea of a "real man" boils down to how well they distance themselves from anything to do with femininity.

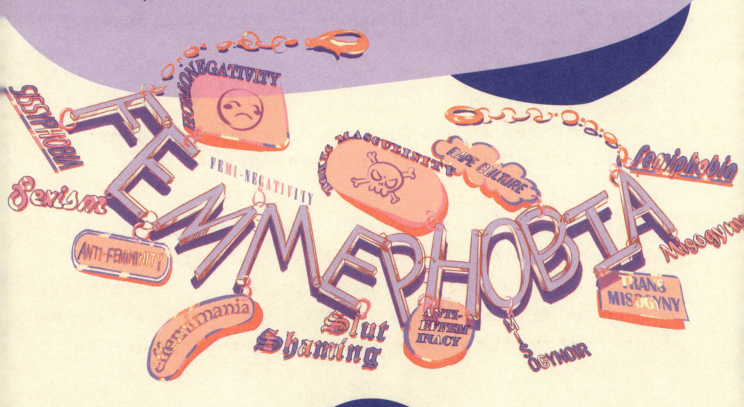

"What feminine part of yourself did you have to destroy in order to survive in this world?"

Alok Vaid-Menon (2017)

SELF-REFLECTION

How would you respond to Alok's question? In what ways have you destroyed, abandoned, or distanced a feminine part of yourself?

_____
_____
_____
_____
_____
_____
_____
_____
_____
_____

In what ways have you made others feel like they needed to "destroy" a feminine part of themselves?

_____
_____
_____
_____
_____
_____
_____
_____
_____
_____
_____
_____
_____
_____
_____

NAMING OUR EXPERIENCES

In what other ways has femmephobia impacted your life?

_____
_____
_____
_____
_____
_____
_____
_____
_____
_____
_____
_____
_____
_____
_____
_____
_____
_____
_____
_____
_____
_____
_____
_____
_____
_____
_____
_____
_____
_____

Communicating the "rules" of Femininity

As we have seen, femmephobia can take many forms, and so can people's experiences of femmephobia. They can range anywhere from what we call "microaggressions" - seemingly small comments/digs related to everyday behaviours and choices, like what people eat or personal grooming - to "macroaggressions," which include bigger things like violence, assault, and even homicide. Whether micro or macro, femmephobia means that we value femininity less and target people who don't follow the "rules" of femininity. These rules or expectations are based on society's narrow definition of femininity, and how well a person seems to fit society's expectations of how they should look or act. At the end of the day, when we treat femininity as something inferior or judge certain expressions of femininity negatively, this is femmephobia.

Some of the everyday ways we may see or experience femmephobia include our food choices (e.g., eating salads versus pork chops), our home décor options (e.g., buying flowers versus mounted deer heads), and our personal grooming (e.g., makeup versus beard trimming/sculpting). In many of these examples, the feminine option is mocked when done by men, and seen as silly when done by women.

Although these experiences may be small, routine parts of our lives, over time, being continuously made fun of, challenged, or ridiculed about what we eat or how we decorate our homes can have a big impact. These seemingly "small experiences" add up throughout the day and over the course of our lives. Not only can they impact how we feel about ourselves and our worth, but they can also place limitations on what we believe we can be and achieve.

Whether it's eating a salad, buying flowers, or moisturizing your skin, we all encounter the pressures of femmephobia regardless of our gender expression, gender identity, sexual orientation, or relationship to femininity.

Where did these "rules" come from?

How did you come to learn that being feminine meant something negative, like being less strong, capable, competent, etc.?

Planting the Seeds

Thinking back to your own family, what are two or three messages you received that planted some of these early seeds of feminine devaluation? These can be intentional or unintentional messages.

_____
_____
_____
_____
_____
_____
_____
_____
_____
_____
_____
_____

For those who are parents, caregivers, or even mentors, think about one or two ways that you may have unintentionally been sending messages that devalue femininity to others.

_____
_____
_____
_____
_____
_____
_____
_____
_____
_____
_____
_____

Limits on Femininity

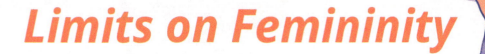

Now that we have a basic understanding of femmephobia, let's talk about how femininity is controlled or regulated!

What are some of the limits we place on "acceptable femininity"? What kinds of femininity do we, or society, see as acceptable? What is unacceptable? For whom?

For whom? Acceptable / OK	For whom? Unacceptable / Not OK

REGULATING FEMININITY

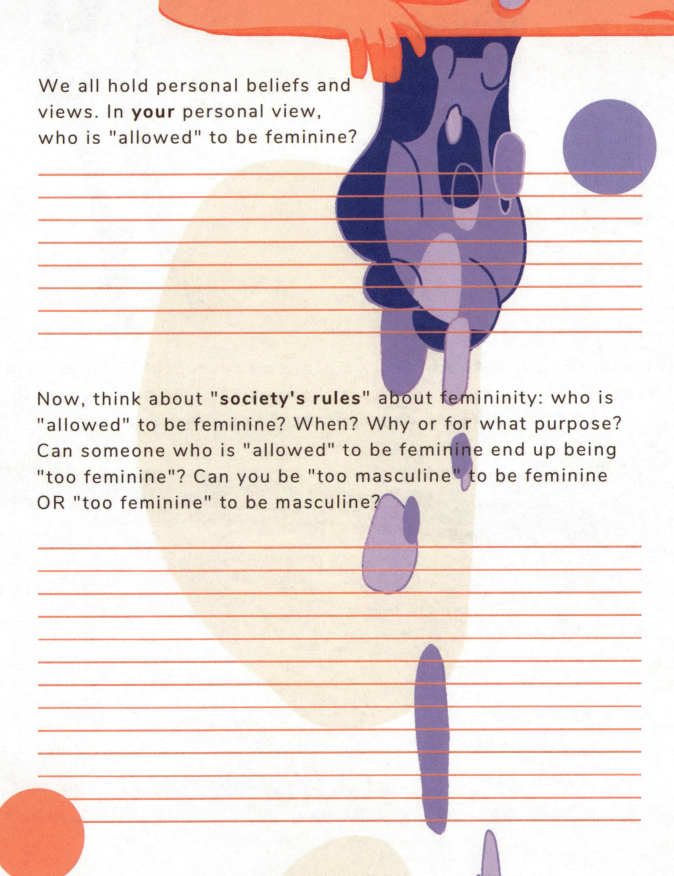

We all hold personal beliefs and views. In **your** personal view, who is "allowed" to be feminine?

_____
_____
_____
_____
_____
_____
_____

Now, think about "**society's rules**" about femininity: who is "allowed" to be feminine? When? Why or for what purpose? Can someone who is "allowed" to be feminine end up being "too feminine"? Can you be "too masculine" to be feminine OR "too feminine" to be masculine?

_____
_____
_____
_____
_____
_____
_____
_____
_____
_____
_____

INTERSECTIONALITY

The "rules" of femininity are not just about the gender binary where we divide gender into man/woman, or about what/where/when we value masculinity over femininity. For example, not showing too much emotion and dressing less "femininely" (i.e., expressing more "masculine-coded" behaviours) might be valued in the workplace for women, but not in other spaces like dinner parties, dances, or dating.

The rules may also change depending on a person's race, age, ethnicity, class, ability, or religion (and so much more!). Each of these parts of people's social identity shapes the "rules" or "expectations" for femininity a bit differently. For example, how we expect girls and women to be feminine is a bit different for a young girl, a young woman, or an older woman, and these rules may further change if she is White or Black, straight or queer, disabled or able-bodied, or of a higher or lower "class."

The way that these parts of our identity shape the rules of femininity is called "intersectionality"(Crenshaw, 1989), meaning that none of us is ever "just one thing"(e.g., woman) – parts of our social identity mesh together (or "intersect") to create a unique experience of any type of oppression or prejudice. So, when we talk about femmephobia (or other kinds of oppression), we also have to think about how race, sexuality, class, and so on can shape the "rules" in different situations or contexts.

Intersectionality encourages us to think about people as a complex mix of identities so there is no "one size fits all" for femininity or any other social identity axis.

INTERSECTIONAL RULES FOR FEMININITY

We've spent a lot of time unpacking your personal and societal "rules" about femininity. Now we ask you to think about the ways that intersections of race, age, dis/ability, class, religion (and so forth) might affect the "rules" for femininity. What sorts of things come to mind for you?

REGULATING FEMININITY THROUGH PATRIARCHAL FEMININITY

"Patriarchal femininity" refers to society's "ideal" version of femininity - a type of femininity that follows the "rules" and "norms" of WHO can be feminine and "HOW."

Patriarchal femininity says that femininity only belongs to White, heterosexual, cisgender, able-bodied women who are passive, thin but curvy, sexually available but not sexually desirous, and who accept being seen as "lesser"-- to name a few characteristics! And, of course, patriarchal femininity sees femininity as being done exclusively for men's attention (and that's partly why people react so negatively to femininity in men).

PATRIARCHAL FEMININITY

- Femininity performed for the male gaze
- Passive
- Normatively White
- Assigned female at birth
- Heterosexual
- Able-bodied
- Oppressive
- Impossible to achieve

FEMME

- Challenges or "fails" to meet the rules of patriarchal femininity
- Femininity not performed for men
- LGBTQ+ identified
- Agentic
- Not necessarily a woman
- Inclusive of diverse ways of being feminine

Femmephobia helps patriarchal femininity to achieve its goal of femininity ONLY existing as this "ideal" version. Through femmephobia, femininity that DOESN'T follow the rules of patriarchal femininity is mocked, ridiculed, and excluded.

Femmes don't "follow the rules," which is why the term "femmephobia" comes from this community and why femmes experience femmephobia.

A FALSE BINARY?

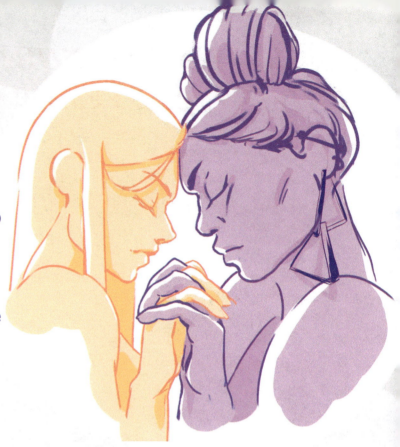

Does this division between patriarchal femininity and femme create a false belief that people and things can only ever be "either/or"? Many of us already know that the world is not so clear-cut between us/them, good/bad, white/black, and so on. These divisions are what some people call a "false binary."

For example, Allen (2022) describes a false binary as only seeing people's experiences "in either/or terms." This sets us up to see a "good/bad" split, where the first one is "privileged and valued," and the second is "oppressed and devalued." But human experiences are really complicated and difficult to categorize neatly into this-or-that – it's often somewhere in-between! So, we need to be careful about not drawing a false (either/or) binary between patriarchal femininity and femme.

Challenging patriarchal femininity is a lot of work and doesn't always feel "liberating." Rejecting or pushing back against "beauty norms," rigid ideas about gender, or assumptions people make about us can be an ongoing and exhausting process, rather than a final destination.

So, instead of seeing femme and patriarchal femininity as arch-enemies, we see femme as a tool for inviting people to think about femininity, and developing a healthier relationship to femininity - a form of femme-inist consciousness raising!

Femme invites people to pick and chose the aspects of femininity they like, and respectfully disregard the rest - a form of DIY femininity!
(Hoskin & Taylor, 2019)

Does femininity have to mean sexually available to men?

Does femininity have to mean woman?

Does femininity have to be oppressive?

Which parts of femininity serve to empower me?

Which do not?

PUTTING A STOP TO FEMMEPHOBIA

We've spent a lot of time thinking about femmephobia, who it affects, and how. Now let's think about **what we can do to reduce femmephobia** in ourselves and in others.

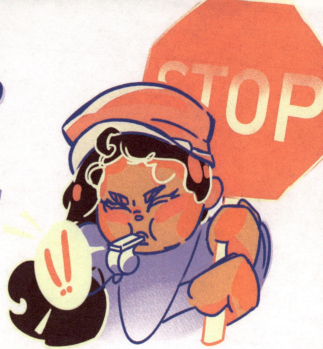

What's one thing you could do when you witness femmephobia?

What's one new way you could embrace your own femininity?

What's one new way you could celebrate femininity in others?

Ask why it's weird • Promote feminine expressions • Support femmes • Identify assumptions • Reconsider assumptions • Be feminine • **Educate** • Call it in • Challenge with love • Challenge assumptions • Make • Encourage femininity • Speak up • Calling it out • Ask why it's funny • Name femmephobia • Challenge other people's assumptions • Challenge stereotypes • Call it out • Challenge our own assumptions • corrections • Interrupt expectations • Value femmes • Name it • Question femmephobia • Acknowledge femmes • Rephrase

Above are some other thoughts on how we can stop femmephobia. Which ones stand out most for you and why?

___

- 49 -

EVERY DAY ACTIVISM

What are some easy steps you can take to reduce femmephobia?

What is the femmephobic stereotype, action, or incident?

What steps can I take to challenge it in the moment?

I've noticed that people often use femininity as the brunt of a joke. For example, a comedy show where a man puts on a dress or makeup, or how we put makeup on pictures of Donald Trump to make fun of him. This sometimes comes up with my friends when they feminize something or someone they want to make fun of.

Question why it is funny, challenge people who make these jokes by asking them to explain why it is funny, reflecting on whether or not the joke would be funny if it involved masculinity. Sometimes just asking people to explain an offensive joke goes a long way!

Reflection to Action: Bystander to Upstander

We've all been a bystander to femmephobia at some point - seeing it around us and not doing anything about it. It can be difficult to be an upstander, someone who defends or protects people who are on the receiving end of femmephobia.

1. What could being a "bystander" to femmephobia look like?

   _____
   _____
   _____
   _____
   _____
   _____
   _____

2. What could being an "upstander" against femmephobia look like?

   _____
   _____
   _____
   _____
   _____
   _____
   _____

How can you move from bystander to upstander? How can you put what you learned in this workbook into action?

_____
_____
_____
_____
_____

Revaluing Femininity

What would happen to femmephobia if we began thinking about femininity differently, and more positively?

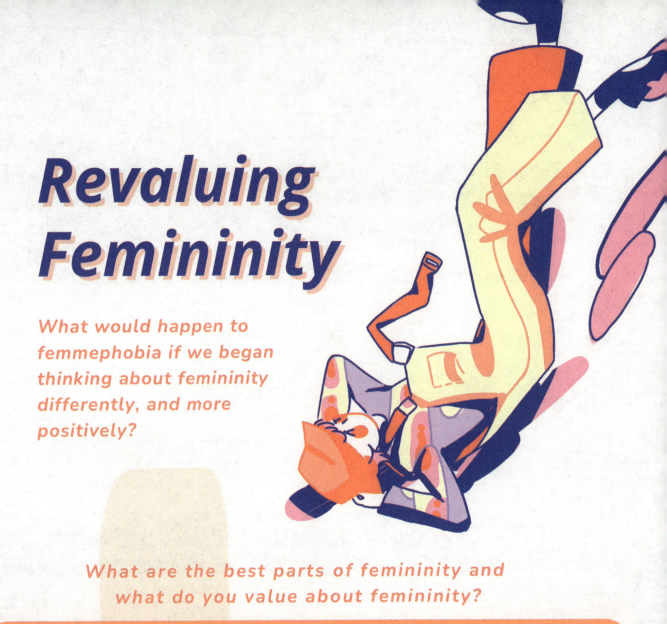

What are the best parts of femininity and what do you value about femininity?

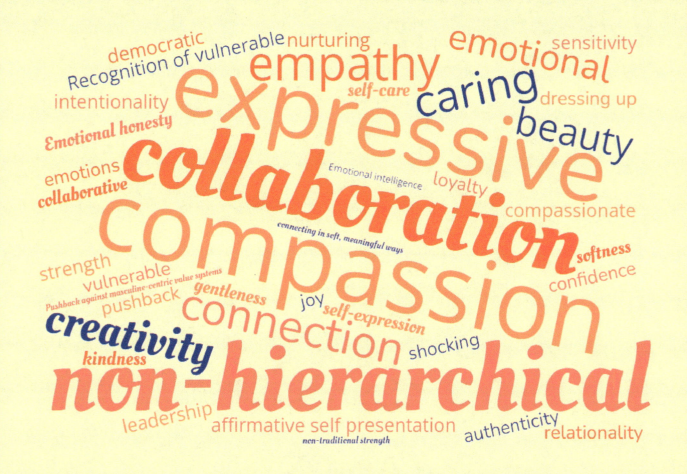

Above are some things that other people value about femininity. Which ones stand out most for you and why?

_____
_____
_____
_____
_____
_____
_____
_____
_____
_____

Revaluing Femininity

What parts of femininity would you like the world to value?

_____
_____
_____
_____

What parts of society would change if we valued these parts of femininity?

_____
_____
_____
_____
_____

Who will this impact?

_____
_____
_____
_____
_____

When we don't value these parts of femininity, who benefits?

_____
_____
_____
_____

Revaluing Femininity

Revaluing femininity could take the form of embracing things like bright and bold styling choices, or not shying away from emotionality and vulnerability. It could also mean challenging the idea that femininity is weak or something to objectify. Regardless of how we personally express gender, revaluing femininity allows us to recognize and embrace ourselves and others more fully since we are all **impacted by femmephobia.**

Women, men, and nonbinary people, of all sexual orientations, whether masculine, feminine, or androgynous, can all experience femmephobia.

Take Aways

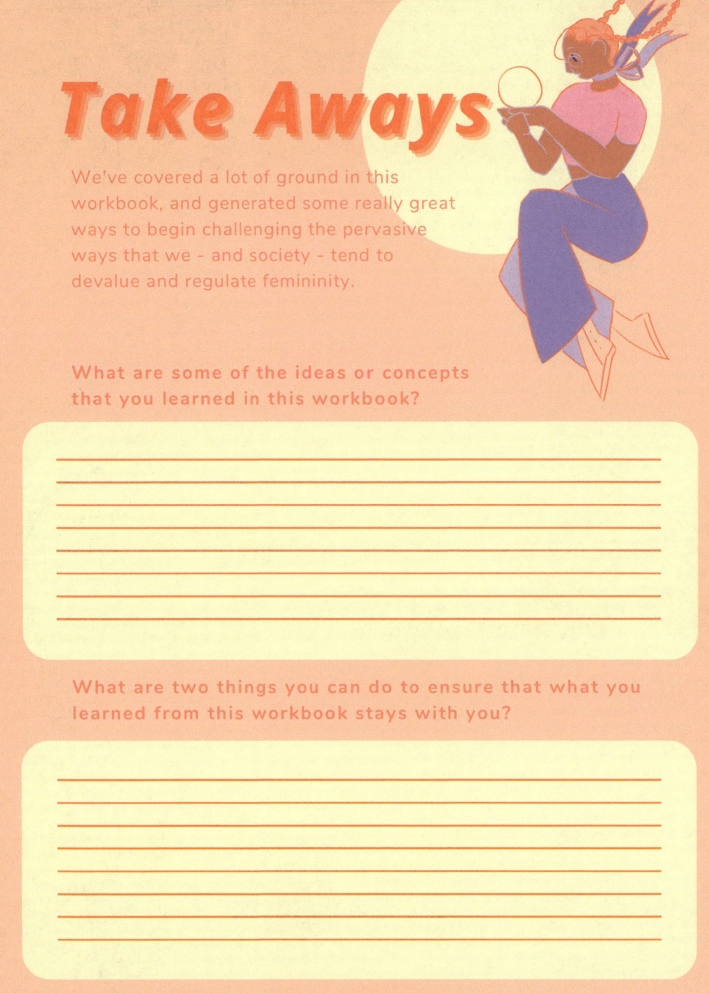

We've covered a lot of ground in this workbook, and generated some really great ways to begin challenging the pervasive ways that we - and society - tend to devalue and regulate femininity.

What are some of the ideas or concepts that you learned in this workbook?

_____
_____
_____
_____
_____
_____
_____
_____

What are two things you can do to ensure that what you learned from this workbook stays with you?

_____
_____
_____
_____
_____
_____
_____

MAYBE YOU LEARNED...

"We all have a relationship with femininity."

"I love thinking about the 'banal' ways that femininity can be challenged."

"I am not a problem that needs to be fixed. I have value and bring a lot to the table just as I am."

"Identifying positive traits that I can recognize in myself, and use it to help me in the future."

"Masculinity is not gender neutral."

"We don't have to kill off part of ourselves to fit other peoples' standards."

"Regardless of your identity or gender expression, you can interrupt femmephobia by celebrating your own femininity and feminine traits."

"Devaluing femininity is playing into the gender binary."

"I think we could all stand to be more feminine - it would be beneficial."

"How femmephobia can impact so many people and across contexts like work, home, and school."

"Femmephobia affects everyone."

Above are some take-aways others have noted. Which ones stand out most for you and why?

_____ _____
_____ _____
_____ _____
_____ _____
_____ _____
_____ _____

As the workbook creators, we hope readers will take away that...

1 — Femmephobia hurts us all.

2 — Femmephobic attitudes support other types of gender-based oppression.

3 — Femininity, like any aspect of identity or expression, is deeply intersectional (i.e., connected to other parts of people's identity, like race, class, ability, and others).

4 — We all have the capacity to have femmephobic beliefs, act in femmephobic ways, and be on the receiving end of femmephobia itself.

5 — We are born into a world of "gender rules" that are so taken-for-granted most of us don't even notice them, let alone question them. We need to begin questioning these rules and the way they limit, restrict, and devalue femininity.

6 — Embracing the value of femininity and encouraging others to do the same are two key ways to challenge femmephobia in ourselves and others.

Letter to Myself

Reflecting on what you've learned in this workbook, what would you say to your past self?

FINAL REFLECTION

As a final reflection, think of three people who would benefit from this workbook and reflect on:

1. _____
2. _____
3. _____

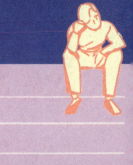

Why you chose them and what they may gain from learning about femmephobia?

_____

How has femmephobia impacted their lives?

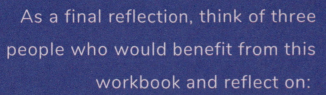

_____

How have their femmephobic views impacted the lives of those around them?

_____

CONTACT INFORMATION

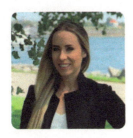

DR. RHEA ASHLEY HOSKIN

- @Femme_Research
- @Femme_inist
- Femme Research
- www.AshleyHoskin.ca

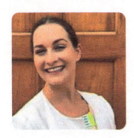

DR. JOCELYNE SCOTT

- @Feminist_Dog_Mom
- jbs036@bucknell.edu

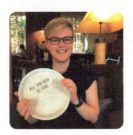

DR. KAREN BLAIR

- @KLBresearch
- @KLBresearch
- www.KLBresearch.com
- KLB Research

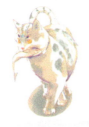

CINDY ZHANG

- LinkedIn: Cynthia (Yu Xin) Zhang
- @glycyerine
- cyn.a.zhang@gmail.com

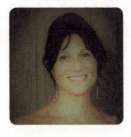

TONI SERAFINI

- tserafini@uwaterloo.ca

RESOURCES & FURTHER READINGS

Allen, K. R. (2022). Feminist theory, method, and praxis: Toward a critical consciousness for family and close relationship scholars. *Journal of Social and Personal Relationships, 40*(3), 899–936.

Blair, K. L., & Hoskin, R. A. (2015). Experiences of femme identity: Coming out, invisibility and femmephobia. *Psychology & Sexuality, 6*(3), 229–244.

Blair, K. L., & Hoskin, R. A. (2016). Contemporary understandings of femme identities and related experiences of discrimination. *Psychology & Sexuality, 7*(2), 101–115.

Brushwood Rose, C., & Camilleri, A. (2002). *Brazen femme: Queering femininity*. Arsenal Pulp.

Burke, J. C. (Ed.). (2009). *Visible: A femmethology (Vol. 1)*. Homofactus Press.

Coyote, I. E., & Sharman, Z. (Eds.). (2011). *Persistence: All ways butch and femme*. Arsenal Pulp.

Crenshaw, K. (1989). Demarginalizing the intersection of race and sex: A Black feminist critique of antidiscrimination doctrine, feminist theory, and antiracist politics. *University of Chicago Legal Forum, 53*(1), 139–167.

Dahl, U. (2012). Turning like a femme: Figuring critical femininity studies. *Nora - Nordic Journal of Feminist and Gender Research, 20*(1), 57–64.

Davies, A. W. J. (2020). "Authentically" effeminate? Bialystok's theorization of authenticity, gay male femmephobia, and personal identity. *Canadian Journal of Family and Youth, 12*(1), 104–123.

Duggan, L., & McHugh, K. (1996). A fem(me)inist manifesto. *Women & Performance: A Journal of Feminist Theory, 8*(2), 153–159.

Erickson, L. (2007). Revealing femmegimp: A sex-positive reflection on sites of shame as sites of resistance for people with disabilities. *Atlantis, 31*(2), 42–52.

Galewski, E. (2005). Figuring the feminist femme. *Women's Studies in Communication, 28*(2), 183–206.

Gomez, J. (1998). Femme erotic independence. In S. R. Munt (Ed.), *Butch/femme: Inside lesbian gender* (pp. 101–108). Cassell.

Gunn, A., Hoskin, R. A., & Blair, K. L. (2021). The new lesbian aesthetic? Exploring gender style among femme, butch and androgynous sexual minority women. *Women's Studies International Forum, 88*, 1-13.

Harris, L., & Crocker, E. (1997). *Femme: Feminists lesbians and bad girls*. Routledge.

Hemmings, C. (1999). Out of sight, out of mind? Theorizing femme narrative. *Sexualities, 2*(4), 451–464.

Hobson, K. (2013). Performative tensions in female drag performances. *Kaleidoscope: A Graduate Journal of Qualitative Communication Research, 12*(4), 35-51.

Hoskin, R. A. (2017a). Femme theory: Refocusing the intersectional lens. *Atlantis: Critical Studies in Gender, Culture & Social Justice, 38*(1), 95–109.

Hoskin, R. A. (2017b). Femme interventions and the proper feminist subject: Critical approaches to decolonizing contemporary Western feminist pedagogies. *Cogent Social Sciences, 3*, 1–17.

Hoskin, R. A. (2019). Femmephobia: The role of anti-femininity and gender policing in LGBTQ + people's experiences of discrimination. *Sex Roles, 81*(11–12), 686–703.

Hoskin, R. A. (2020). "Femininity? It's the aesthetic of subordination": Examining femmephobia, the gender binary, and experiences of oppression among sexual and gender minorities. *Archives of Sexual Behavior, 49*(7), 2319-2339.

Hoskin, R. A. (2021a). Can femme be theory? Exploring the epistemological and methodological possibilities of femme. *Journal of Lesbian Studies, 25*(1), 1-17.

Hoskin, R. A. (Ed.). (2021b). *Feminizing theory: Making space for femme theory*. Routledge.

Hoskin, R. A., & Hirschfeld, K. L. (2018). Beyond aesthetics: A femme manifesto. *Atlantis: Critical Studies in Gender, Culture & Social Justice, 39*(1), 85–87.

Hoskin, R. A., & Taylor, A. (2019). Femme resistance: The femme-inine art of failure. *Psychology & Sexuality, 10*(4), 281–300

Hoskin, R. A., & Blair, K. L. (2021). Critical femininities: a 'new' approach to gender theory. *Psychology & Sexuality, 13*(1), 1-8.

Hoskin, R. A., & Serafini, T. (2023). Critically feminizing family science: Using femme theory to generate novel approaches for the study of families and relationships. *Journal of Family Theory & Review, 15*(2), 292-312.

Hoskin, R. A., & Whiley, L. A. (2023). Femme-toring: Leveraging critical femininities and femme theory to cultivate alternative approaches to mentoring. *Gender, Work & Organization*, 1-17.

Kattari, S. K., & Beltran, R. (2019). Twice blessed: An Auto-archaeology of femme crip (in)visibility. *Departures in Critical Qualitative Research, 8*(3), 8–28.

Keeling, K. (2007). *The witch's flight: The cinematic, the black femme and the image of common sense*. Duke University Press.

Kennedy, E. L., & Davis, M. D. (1993). *Boots of leather, slippers of gold: The history of a lesbian community.* Routledge/Penguin.

Lev, A. I. (2008). More than surface tension: Femmes in families. *Journal of Lesbian Studies, 12*(2–3), 127–143.

Levitt, H., Gerrish, E. A., & Hiestand, K. R. (2003). The misunderstood gender: A model of modern femme identity. *Sex Roles, 48*(3–4), 99–113.

Lewis, S. F. (2012). "Everything I know about being femme I learned from Sula" or toward a Black femme-inist criticism. *Trans-Scripts, 2*, 100–125.

Matheson, L., Ortiz, D. L., Hoskin, R. A., Holmberg, D., & Blair, K. L. (2021). The feminine target: Gender expression in same-sex relationships as a predictor of experiences with public displays of affection. *The Canadian Journal of Human Sexuality, 30*(2), 205-218.

McCann, H. (2018). Beyond the visible: Rethinking femininity through the femme assemblage. *European Journal of Women's Studies, 25*(3), 278–292.

McCann, H., & Killen, G. (2019). Femininity isn't femme: Appearance and the contradictory space of queer femme belongings. In A. Tsalapatanis, M. Bruce, D. Bissel, H. Keane (Eds.), *Social beings, future belongings: Reimagining the social* (pp. 135–147). Routledge.

McCann, H. (2020). Is there anything "toxic" about femininity? The rigid femininities that keep us locked in. *Psychology & Sexuality, 13*(1), 1–14.

Miller, B., & Behm-Morawitz, E. (2016). "Masculine Guys Only": The effects of femmephobic mobile dating application profiles on partner selection for men who have sex with men. *Computers in Human Behavior*, 62, 176-185.

Nestle, J. (Ed.). (1992). *The persistent desire: A femme-butch reader.* Alyson Books.

Samuels, E. (2003). My body, my closet: Invisible disability and the limits of coming-out discourse. *GLQ: A Journal of Lesbian and Gay Studies, 9*(1–2), 233–255.

Schwartz, A. (2018). Locating femme theory online. *First Monday, 23*(7).

Schwartz, A. (2020). Radical vulnerability: Selfies as a Femme-inine mode of resistance. *Psychology & Sexuality, 13*(1), 1–14.

Scott, J. B. (2020). What do glitter, pointe shoes, & plastic drumsticks have in common? Using femme theory to consider the reclamation of disciplinary beauty/body practices. *The Journal of Lesbian Studies, 25*(1), 36–52.

Scott, J. B. (2021). Negotiating relationships with powerfulness: Using femme theory to resist masculinist pressures on feminist femininities. *Psychology & Sexuality, 13*(1), 1–10.

Serano, J. (2007). *Whipping girl: A transsexual woman on sexism and the scapegoating of femininity*. Seal Press.

Serano, J. (2013). *Excluded: Making feminist and queer movements more inclusive*. Seal Press.

Shelton, P. (2018). Reconsidering femme identity: On centering trans* counterculture and conceptualizing trans*femme theory. *Journal of Black Sexuality and Relationships, 5*(1), 21–41.

Story, K. A. (2017). Fear of a Black femme: The existential conundrum of embodying a Black femme identity while being a professor of Black, queer, and feminist studies. *Journal of Lesbian Studies, 21*(4), 407–419.

Taylor, A. (2018). "Flabulously" femme: Queer fat femme women's identities and experiences. *Journal of Lesbian Studies, 22*(4), 459–481.

Taylor, A. (2020). "But where are the dates?" Dating as a central site of fat femme marginalisation in queer communities. *Psychology & Sexuality, 13*(1), 57-68.

Tinsley, O. M. (2015). Femmes of color, femmes de couleur: Theorizing Black queer femininity through Chauvet's La Danse sur le Volcan. *Yale French Studies, 128*, 131–145.

Vaid-Menon, A. (2017). *Femme in public*. Alok Vaid-Menon: Self-Published.

VanNewkirk, R. (2006). "Gee, I didn't get that vibe from you": Articulating my own version of a femme lesbian existence. *Journal of Lesbian Studies, 10*(1–2), 73–85.

Volcano, D. L., & Dahl, U. (2008). *Femmes of power: Exploding queer femininities*. Serpent's Tail.

Walker, L. (2012). The future of femme: Notes on ageing, femininity, and gender theory. *Sexualities, 15*(7), 795–814.

Whiley, L. A., Stutterheim, S., & Grandy, G. (2020). Breastfeeding, 'tainted' love, and femmephobia: Containing the 'dirty' performances of embodied femininity. *Psychology & Sexuality, 13*(1), 101–114.

Extra Notes

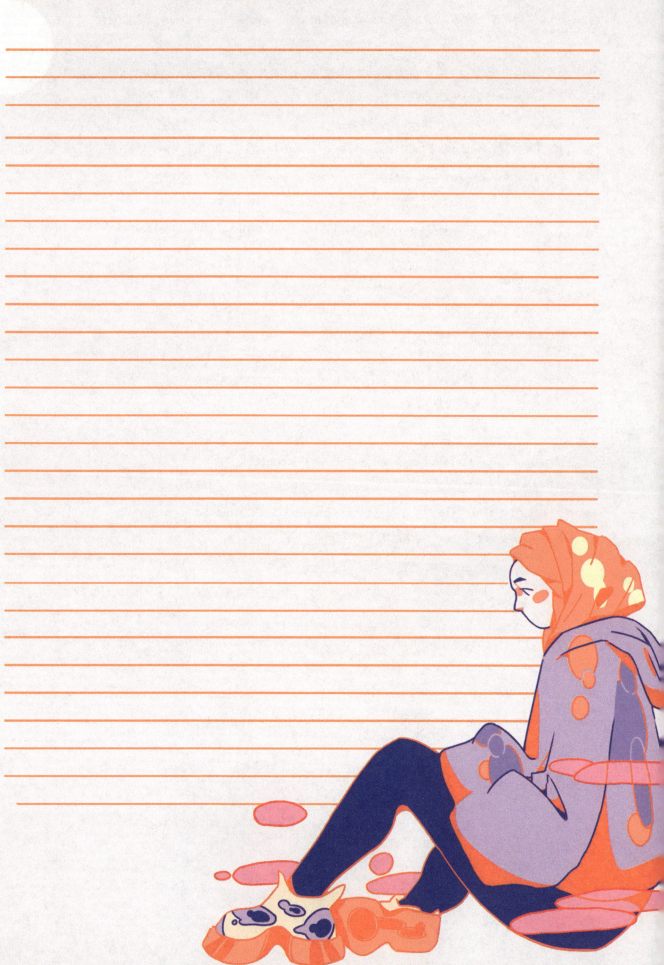

Extra Notes

This workbook was created by Drs. Rhea Ashley Hoskin, Toni Serafini, Jocelyne Scott, & Karen Blair (2023).

Illustrated by Cindy Zhang

We welcome feedback for future editions.

The Femmephobia 101 Workbook

www.femmephobia.com

Support for the creation of this workbook was provided by the University of Waterloo's AMTD Global Talent Postdoctoral Fellowship Program and the Social Sciences and Humanities Research Council of Canada.

 Social Sciences and Humanities Research Council of Canada   Conseil de recherches en sciences humaines du Canada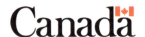

Recommended Reading

Defending Against Attack
"The Shōtōkan Way"
By Frank Nezhadpournia

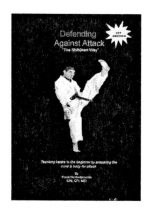

Defending Against Attack
For Women (2nd Edition)
By Frank Nezhadpournia

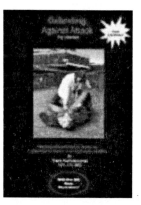

Defending Against Attack
"The Complete Guide" DVD
By Frank Nezhadpournia & Mark Lawn
Featuring Michelle Ericsson

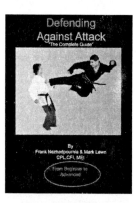

Advanced Shotokan
By Frank Nezhadpournia

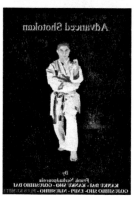

Published by Actikarate Ltd
Distributed by Gazelle Book Services Limited,
White Cross Mills, Hightown,
LANCASTER LA1 4XS, UK
Website: www.gazellebooks.co.uk **Email:** sales@gazellebooks.co.uk
Distributors to the Martial Arts Trade: TSA Martial Arts, Access Storage Building, 1A Neptune Road, Harrow, Middlesex, HA1 4HY.

Artists who have helped me along my path!
'You give without wanting and support without hesitating!'

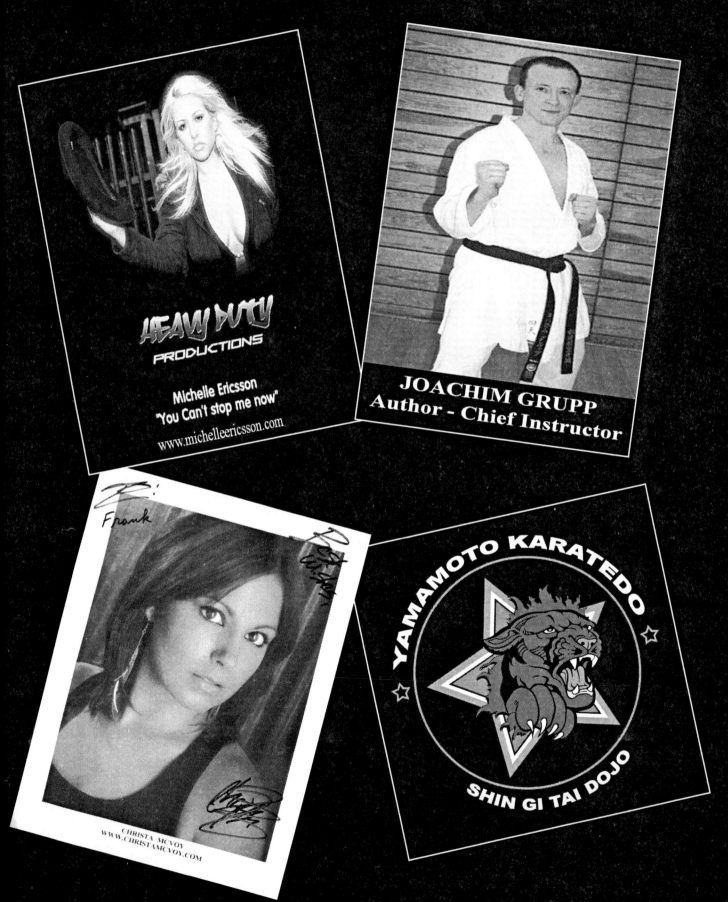